LOW FODMAP ENDOMETRIOSIS COOKBOOK

COOKBOOK

2024

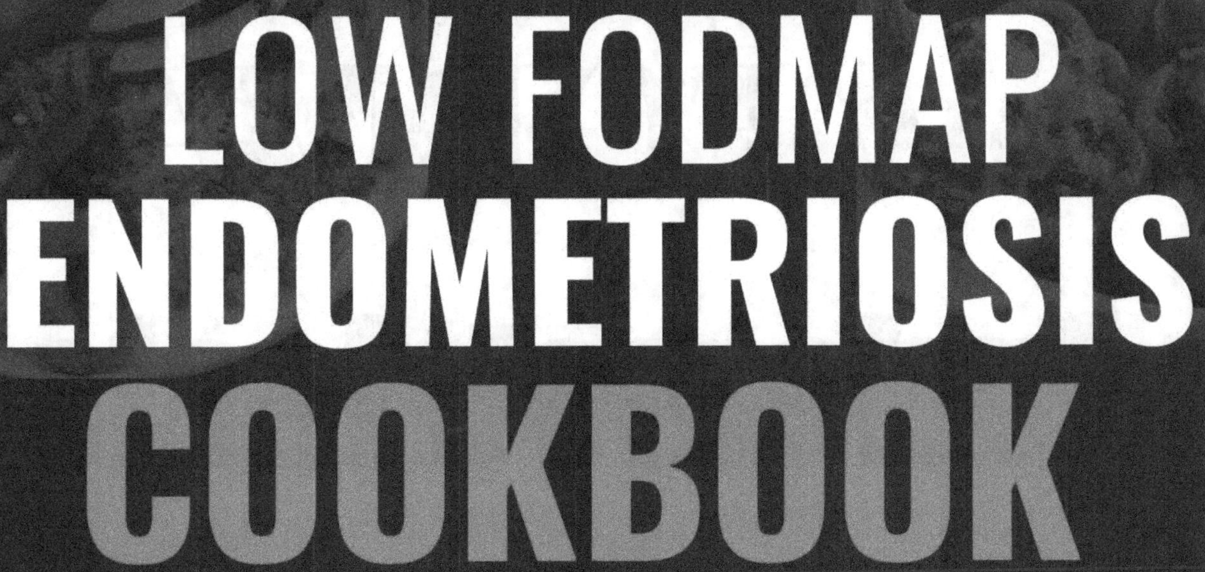

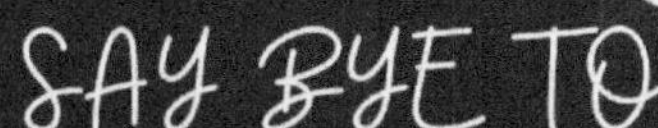

PELVIC PAIN, PAINFUL MENSTRUATION, PAINFUL INTERCOURSE, INFERTILITY, BACK PAIN, FATIGUE, BLOATING, PAINFUL URINATION

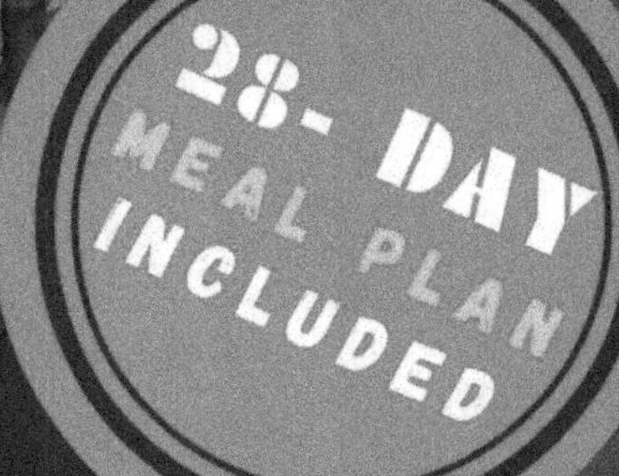

Low FODMAP

Endometriosis

Cookbook

Nutrient-Rich Recipes and 28-Day Meal Plan for Digestive Wellness, Bloating Relief, Abdominal Comfort, Pelvic Pain, Dysmenorrhea Management, Improved Fertility, and More"

Judy Kelly

Table of Contents

Introduction

- Understanding Endometriosis

Endometriosis is a complex and often painful medical condition that affects the tissue lining the uterus, known as the endometrium. In this condition, tissue similar to the lining of the uterus grows outside the uterus, leading to a range of symptoms and potential complications. While the exact cause of endometriosis remains unclear, several factors contribute to its development.

1. Common Symptoms:
   - Pelvic Pain: One of the primary symptoms is pelvic pain, ranging from mild discomfort to severe, debilitating pain.
   - Menstrual Irregularities: Women with endometriosis may experience irregular periods, heavy menstrual flow, or spotting between periods.
   - Painful Intercourse: Pain during or after sexual intercourse is a common complaint among individuals with endometriosis.
   - Infertility: Endometriosis can be associated with fertility issues, making it challenging for some women to conceive.

2. Diagnostic Challenges:
   - Diagnosing endometriosis can be challenging as symptoms can vary widely, and they may overlap with other conditions.
   - Laparoscopy, a minimally invasive surgical procedure, is often necessary for a definitive diagnosis by visualizing and confirming the presence of endometrial tissue outside the uterus.

3. Impact on Quality of Life:
   - Beyond the physical symptoms, endometriosis can significantly impact a person's emotional well-being and quality of life.
   - Chronic pain and the uncertainty surrounding fertility can contribute to anxiety, depression, and stress.

4. Possible Causes and Risk Factors:

- The exact cause of endometriosis remains unclear, but several factors may contribute, including genetics, hormonal imbalances, and immune system dysfunction.
- Women with a family history of endometriosis are at a higher risk, suggesting a genetic component.

5. Treatment Approaches:
- Endometriosis management often involves a combination of medical and surgical interventions.
- Pain relief medications, hormonal therapies, and, in some cases, surgery may be recommended to alleviate symptoms and improve quality of life.

6. Lifestyle and Dietary Considerations:
- Some individuals find relief from symptoms by adopting a low FODMAP diet, which restricts certain types of fermentable carbohydrates that can contribute to gastrointestinal symptoms associated with endometriosis.

7. Holistic Support:
- Managing endometriosis requires a holistic approach that includes not only medical interventions but also lifestyle modifications, emotional support, and nutritional strategies.

Understanding endometriosis is crucial for those affected and their support networks. By raising awareness and fostering a deeper understanding of this condition, we can work towards better support, early detection, and improved management strategies for individuals living with endometriosis.

- The Low FODMAP Approach

The Low FODMAP (Fermentable Oligosaccharides, Disaccharides, Monosaccharides, and Polyols) diet is gaining recognition as a valuable approach in managing the symptoms of endometriosis. This dietary strategy focuses on reducing the intake of certain types of carbohydrates that are poorly absorbed in the small intestine and can lead to symptoms such as bloating, gas, and abdominal discomfort. Here's an overview of the key elements of the Low FODMAP approach in the context of endometriosis management:

1. FODMAPs Defined:
   - Oligosaccharides: Found in foods like wheat, onions, and garlic.
   - Disaccharides: Includes lactose found in dairy products.
   - Monosaccharides: Includes fructose found in some fruits.
   - Polyols: Found in certain fruits, vegetables, and artificial sweeteners.

2. Reducing Fermentable Carbohydrates:
   - The primary goal of the Low FODMAP diet is to limit the intake of fermentable carbohydrates that can cause digestive symptoms.
   - This approach involves avoiding or minimizing high FODMAP foods during specific phases of the diet.

3. Identification and Elimination:
   - Individuals typically start with an elimination phase where high FODMAP foods are restricted for a specified period.
   - This phase helps identify specific triggers that may be contributing to symptoms.

4. Reintroduction Phase:
   - Following the elimination phase, certain FODMAP-containing foods are systematically reintroduced to identify which ones can be tolerated without causing symptoms.
   - This phase helps create a personalized and sustainable long-term diet plan.

5. Potential Benefits for Endometriosis:
   - Some individuals with endometriosis report improvements in gastrointestinal symptoms, including bloating and abdominal discomfort, through the Low FODMAP approach.
   - It may also help in managing dysmenorrhea (painful menstruation) and other associated symptoms.

6. Considerations for Nutrient-Rich Choices:
   - While restricting certain FODMAPs, it's essential to prioritize nutrient-rich, well-balanced foods to ensure adequate nutrition.
   - Incorporating a variety of fruits, vegetables, lean proteins, and whole grains that are low in FODMAPs is crucial for overall health.

7. Consultation with a Healthcare Professional:
   - Before starting the Low FODMAP diet, individuals, especially those with endometriosis, should consult with a healthcare professional or a registered dietitian.
   - Personalized guidance can ensure that the diet is tailored to individual needs and nutritional requirements.

8. Integration into Endometriosis Management:
   - The Low FODMAP approach should be seen as part of a comprehensive strategy for managing endometriosis symptoms, including medical interventions, lifestyle modifications, and emotional support.

By understanding and implementing the Low FODMAP approach carefully, individuals with endometriosis may find relief from certain gastrointestinal symptoms, contributing to an overall improvement in their quality of life. It's crucial to approach this dietary strategy with guidance from healthcare professionals to ensure its effectiveness and sustainability.

- How This Cookbook Can Help

The "Low FODMAP Endometriosis Cookbook" is designed as a comprehensive resource to support individuals in managing their endometriosis symptoms through a targeted dietary approach. Here's how this cookbook can be a valuable tool for individuals seeking relief and improved well-being:

1. Understanding Endometriosis:
   - The cookbook begins with an informative section on understanding endometriosis. It provides readers with insights into the condition, its symptoms, and the impact on daily life. This foundational knowledge helps create awareness and a sense of empowerment.

2. Low FODMAP Approach:
   - Clearly explains the Low FODMAP approach, breaking down the types of fermentable carbohydrates to be restricted during specific phases. This information serves as a guide for readers looking to implement this dietary strategy effectively.

3. Practical Kitchen Essentials:
   - Offers guidance on setting up a Low FODMAP-friendly kitchen. This includes a list of essential ingredients, tools, and equipment to make the cooking process seamless and enjoyable.

4. Nutrient-Rich Recipes:
   - Presents a diverse range of nutrient-rich recipes tailored to the Low FODMAP framework. The recipes are carefully crafted to minimize high FODMAP ingredients while maximizing flavor, ensuring that individuals with endometriosis can enjoy delicious meals without triggering symptoms.

5. 28-Day Meal Plan:
   - Provides a structured 28-day meal plan, offering a week-by-week guide to help individuals plan their meals effectively. This not only saves time but also ensures a balanced and varied diet throughout the month.

6. Symptom Management:

- Dedicated chapters offer practical advice on tailoring the diet to manage specific symptoms associated with endometriosis, such as pelvic pain, bloating, and dysmenorrhea. This targeted guidance helps individuals address their unique challenges.

7. Improved Fertility and Nutrition:

- Recognizes the link between nutrition and fertility in the context of endometriosis. The cookbook includes insights and recipes that support fertility and overall reproductive health through a nutrient-dense and well-balanced diet.

8. Tips for Success:

- Offers practical tips for successfully incorporating Low FODMAP principles into daily life. This section addresses common challenges, provides motivational strategies, and encourages readers to enjoy the journey toward better digestive wellness.

9. Comprehensive Resource:

- Serves as a comprehensive resource by including a conclusion that highlights the path to wellness and a list of further support resources. This ensures that readers have ongoing assistance and access to additional information beyond the cookbook.

10. Accessibility and Enjoyment:

- Emphasizes the importance of making the Low FODMAP approach accessible and enjoyable. The cookbook aims to dispel any misconceptions about restrictive diets by showcasing a variety of flavorful and satisfying recipes.

By combining education, practical advice, and a collection of delicious recipes, the "Low FODMAP Endometriosis Cookbook" becomes a valuable tool for individuals navigating the challenges of endometriosis. It empowers readers to take control of their diet, manage symptoms effectively, and work towards improved digestive wellness and overall well-being.

Chapter 1: Getting Started

- Kitchen Essentials for a Low FODMAP KitchenSetting up a Low FODMAP kitchen requires thoughtful consideration and careful planning to ensure that the necessary tools and ingredients are readily available. Here's a list of kitchen essentials for a Low FODMAP kitchen:

1. Pantry Staples:
   - Gluten-free flours (such as rice flour, tapioca flour, or cornmeal)
   - Low FODMAP sweeteners (e.g., maple syrup, sugar, or stevia)
   - Olive oil or other Low FODMAP cooking oils
   - Herbs and spices (rosemary, thyme, oregano, basil, cumin, etc.)
   - Low FODMAP broth or stock (check labels for garlic and onion content)

2. Fresh Produce:
   - Green leafy vegetables (kale, spinach, lettuce)
   - Bell peppers
   - Carrots
   - Zucchini
   - Cucumber
   - Tomatoes (without excess seeds)
   - Fresh herbs (parsley, cilantro)

3. Protein Sources:
   - Fresh or frozen poultry (chicken or turkey)
   - Fresh or canned fish (salmon, tuna, or cod)
   - Eggs
   - Firm tofu
   - Tempeh
   - Plain, unprocessed meats (beef or pork)

4. Dairy Alternatives:
   - Lactose-free milk or plant-based milk (almond, rice, or coconut)
   - Lactose-free or hard cheeses
   - Lactose-free or plant-based yogurt

5. Grains and Carbohydrates:
  - Quinoa
  - Rice (white or brown)
  - Gluten-free pasta or noodles
  - Oats (gluten-free)
  - Polenta or cornmeal

6. Low FODMAP Baking Supplies:
  - Gluten-free baking powder
  - Gluten-free baking soda
  - Xanthan gum (for gluten-free baking)
  - Dark chocolate (without high FODMAP ingredients)

7. Kitchen Tools:
  - High-quality knives for chopping vegetables and meat
  - Cutting boards (preferably designated for Low FODMAP foods)
  - Non-stick cookware
  - Strainer or colander for draining pasta or washing vegetables
  - Measuring cups and spoons
  - Mixing bowls
  - Blender or food processor

8. Low FODMAP Sauces and Condiments:
  - Soy sauce (gluten-free)
  - Dijon mustard
  - Mayonnaise (without high FODMAP ingredients)
  - Olive tapenade
  - Vinegars (balsamic, red or white wine vinegar)
  - Tomato paste (in moderation)

9. Storage Containers:
  - Airtight containers for storing leftovers
    - Mason jars for meal prepping and storing homemade sauces or dressings

10. Reading Materials:
   - The Monash University Low FODMAP Diet app or printed FODMAP food lists for reference
   - A reliable Low FODMAP cookbook or guide for recipe inspiration and guidance

Remember to check ingredient labels for hidden sources of FODMAPs and be cautious with pre-packaged items. Having a well-equipped Low FODMAP kitchen makes it easier to follow the dietary guidelines and prepare delicious, symptom-friendly meals.

Understanding Nutrient-Rich Ingredients

Understanding nutrient-rich ingredients is essential when following a dietary approach like the Low FODMAP diet for managing endometriosis. It ensures that individuals receive essential nutrients while minimizing the intake of fermentable carbohydrates. Here's a guide to nutrient-rich ingredients suitable for a Low FODMAP diet:

1. Lean Proteins:
   - Poultry: Skinless chicken and turkey are excellent sources of lean protein.
   - Fish: Salmon, cod, and tuna provide omega-3 fatty acids and protein.
   - Eggs: A versatile and nutrient-dense protein source.

2. Low FODMAP Vegetables:
   - Leafy Greens: Spinach, kale, and Swiss chard are rich in vitamins and minerals.
   - Zucchini: A versatile and low-calorie vegetable.
   - Carrots: Provide beta-carotene, an antioxidant.
   - Bell Peppers: Packed with vitamin C.
   - Cucumber: Hydrating and low in FODMAPs.

3. Gluten-Free Grains:
   - Quinoa: A complete protein and rich in fiber.
   - Rice: Both white and brown rice are low FODMAP options.

- Oats: Ensure they are labeled gluten-free for those sensitive to gluten.
- Polenta: A good source of complex carbohydrates.

4. Low FODMAP Fruits:
  - Berries: Blueberries, strawberries, and raspberries are rich in antioxidants.
  - Bananas: Provide potassium and are a low FODMAP fruit.
  - Cantaloupe: A hydrating and nutrient-dense melon.

5. Lactose-Free or Dairy Alternatives:
  - Lactose-Free Milk: A source of calcium and vitamin D.
  - Lactose-Free Yogurt: Provides probiotics and protein.
  - Hard Cheeses: Parmesan, cheddar, and Swiss are low in lactose.

6. Nuts and Seeds:
  - Almonds: A good source of healthy fats and vitamin E.
  - Pumpkin Seeds: Rich in magnesium and zinc.
  - Chia Seeds: Provide omega-3 fatty acids and fiber.

7. Cooking Oils:
  - Olive Oil: A heart-healthy oil rich in monounsaturated fats.
  - Canola Oil: Low in FODMAPs and versatile for cooking.

8. Herbs and Spices:
  - Basil: Adds flavor without FODMAPs.
  - Cilantro: A fresh herb that enhances taste.
  - Turmeric: Known for its anti-inflammatory properties.

9. Gluten-Free Baking Ingredients:
  - Rice Flour: A common gluten-free alternative for baking.
  - Potato Starch: Adds moisture to gluten-free baked goods.
  - Baking Powder (GF): Essential for gluten-free baking.

10. Low FODMAP Sweeteners:
  - Maple Syrup: A natural sweetener.

- Sugar: White or brown sugar in moderation.
- Stevia: A low-calorie sweetener derived from the Stevia plant.

11. Seafood:
  - Shrimp: A low-fat protein source.
  - Scallops: Rich in protein and low in FODMAPs.

Understanding and incorporating these nutrient-rich ingredients into your Low FODMAP kitchen can contribute to a well-balanced and nourishing diet. It's important to consult with a healthcare professional or a registered dietitian to ensure that individual nutritional needs are met while following the Low FODMAP approach.

Tips for Effective Meal Planning

Effective meal planning is a key component of successfully implementing the Low FODMAP approach for managing endometriosis. Here are some tips to help you plan and prepare meals that are not only symptom-friendly but also delicious and nutritionally balanced:

1. Familiarize Yourself with Low FODMAP Foods:
  - Understand the list of Low FODMAP foods and those to be avoided. Utilize resources like the Monash University Low FODMAP Diet app or printed FODMAP food lists for reference.

2. Plan Balanced Meals:
  - Ensure each meal includes a balance of protein, carbohydrates, and healthy fats to provide sustained energy and nutrients.
  - Incorporate a variety of colors and textures by including a mix of vegetables, proteins, and grains.

3. Batch Cooking:
  - Prepare large batches of Low FODMAP recipes that can be portioned and stored for later use. This saves time and ensures you have readily available meals during busy days.

4. Create a Weekly Menu:
   - Plan your meals for the week ahead. This helps in organizing your grocery shopping and ensures that you have all the necessary ingredients on hand.

5. Utilize Leftovers:
   - Plan meals that can easily be repurposed into leftovers for the next day's lunch or dinner. This reduces cooking time and minimizes food waste.

6. Keep It Simple:
   - Choose recipes with simple and readily available ingredients to make meal preparation more manageable.
   - Consider recipes that require minimal cooking time, especially on busy days.

7. Grocery Shopping Tips:
   - Stick to your shopping list to avoid impulse purchases.
   - Shop for fresh produce, proteins, and pantry staples first before exploring other aisles.

8. Label and Organize:
   - Label your ingredients with their FODMAP content to make meal planning and cooking more straightforward.
   - Organize your pantry and refrigerator to easily locate Low FODMAP ingredients.

9. Experiment with Flavors:
   - Use herbs, spices, and low FODMAP condiments to add flavor to your meals without triggering symptoms.
   - Experiment with different seasoning combinations to keep your meals interesting.

10. Consider Portion Sizes:
   - Pay attention to portion sizes, as some individuals may be sensitive to larger quantities of certain Low FODMAP foods.

- Use measuring tools to ensure accurate portions, especially during the elimination and reintroduction phases.

11. Plan for Snacks:
   - Have Low FODMAP snacks readily available to prevent reaching for high FODMAP options when hungry between meals.
   - Pre-portion snacks for convenient grab-and-go options.

12. Stay Hydrated:
   - Include plenty of hydrating options such as water, herbal teas, and infused water in your meal plan.

13. Be Flexible:
   - Be open to adapting your meal plan based on how you feel and any changes in your schedule.
   - Adjust portion sizes and ingredients based on personal tolerance levels.

14. Seek Professional Guidance:
   - Consult with a registered dietitian or healthcare professional for personalized advice and support in creating a meal plan tailored to your individual needs.

Effective meal planning can make a significant difference in managing endometriosis symptoms while following the Low FODMAP approach. It allows for greater control over your diet, ensuring that you enjoy flavorful and nourishing meals that support your overall well-being.

Chapter 2: Breakfasts

1. Energizing Quinoa Breakfast Bowl

Ingredients:
- 1 cup cooked quinoa
- 1/2 cup strawberries, sliced
- 1/4 cup blueberries
- 1 tablespoon chia seeds
- 1 tablespoon slivered almonds
- 1 tablespoon maple syrup (optional)
- Lactose-free yogurt (optional, for serving)

Instructions:
1. In a bowl, combine cooked quinoa, sliced strawberries, blueberries, chia seeds, and slivered almonds.
2. Drizzle with maple syrup if desired for added sweetness.
3. Optional: Serve with a dollop of lactose-free yogurt on top.
4. Mix well and enjoy this nutrient-rich quinoa breakfast bowl.

2. Blueberry Almond Smoothie

Ingredients:
- 1 cup almond milk
- 1/2 cup blueberries (fresh or frozen)
- 1 tablespoon almond butter
- 1 tablespoon chia seeds
- Ice cubes (optional)
- Lactose-free yogurt (optional, for added creaminess)

Instructions:
1. In a blender, combine almond milk, blueberries, almond butter, and chia seeds.
2. Optional: Add a handful of ice cubes for a chilled smoothie.
3. If desired, include a scoop of lactose-free yogurt for extra creaminess.

4. Blend until smooth and pour into a glass. Enjoy this refreshing and nutritious blueberry almond smoothie.

3. Scrambled Tofu with Spinach and Tomatoes

Ingredients:
- 1/2 cup firm tofu, crumbled
- 1 cup fresh spinach, chopped
- 1/2 cup cherry tomatoes, halved
- 1 tablespoon olive oil
- Salt and pepper to taste
- Fresh herbs (such as parsley or chives) for garnish

Instructions:
1. Heat olive oil in a non-stick skillet over medium heat.
2. Add crumbled tofu to the skillet and cook for 2-3 minutes until it starts to brown.
3. Stir in chopped spinach and halved cherry tomatoes.
4. Cook for an additional 3-4 minutes until the vegetables are wilted and tomatoes are slightly softened.
5. Season with salt and pepper to taste.
6. Garnish with fresh herbs and serve this flavorful scrambled tofu with spinach and tomatoes.

4. Lemon Herb Grilled Chicken Salad

Ingredients:
- 1 boneless, skinless chicken breast
- Mixed salad greens (lettuce, spinach, arugula)
- Cherry tomatoes, halved
- Cucumber, sliced
- Olive oil
- Lemon juice
- Dried herbs (rosemary, thyme, oregano)
- Salt and pepper to taste

Instructions:
1. Marinate chicken in olive oil, lemon juice, dried herbs, salt, and pepper.
2. Grill the chicken until fully cooked.
3. Slice the grilled chicken and arrange it over a bed of mixed salad greens.
4. Add cherry tomatoes and cucumber slices.
5. Drizzle with a little more olive oil and lemon juice.
6. Toss the salad gently and serve.

5. Quinoa and Roasted Vegetable Buddha Bowl

Ingredients:
- Cooked quinoa
- Zucchini, sliced
- Bell peppers, sliced
- Carrots, julienned
- Olive oil
- Cumin and paprika for seasoning
- Fresh cilantro for garnish
- Optional: Grilled chicken or tofu for added protein

Instructions:
1. Toss sliced vegetables in olive oil and season with cumin and paprika.
2. Roast the vegetables until they are tender and slightly caramelized.
3. Assemble the Buddha bowl by placing a serving of quinoa in a bowl.
4. Top with roasted vegetables and your choice of protein.
5. Garnish with fresh cilantro and serve.

6. Zucchini Noodles with Pesto and Cherry Tomatoes

Ingredients:
- Zucchini, spiralized into noodles
- Cherry tomatoes, halved
- Pesto sauce (made with basil, pine nuts, Parmesan, olive oil)
- Salt and pepper to taste
- Optional: Grated Parmesan for topping

Instructions:
1. Spiralize zucchini into noodle shapes.
2. In a pan, sauté zucchini noodles until just tender.
3. Mix in pesto sauce and cherry tomatoes.
4. Season with salt and pepper to taste.
5. Optional: Top with grated Parmesan before serving.

7. Baked Salmon with Dill and Lemon

Ingredients:
- Salmon fillets
- Fresh dill, chopped
- Lemon slices
- Olive oil
- Salt and pepper to taste

Instructions:
1. Preheat the oven to 375°F (190°C).
2. Place salmon fillets on a baking sheet.
3. Drizzle with olive oil and sprinkle with fresh dill, salt, and pepper.
4. Top each fillet with lemon slices.
5. Bake for 15-20 minutes or until the salmon flakes easily with a fork.

8. Eggplant and Chickpea Curry

Ingredients:
- Eggplant, diced
- Canned chickpeas, drained and rinsed
- Coconut milk
- Curry powder
- Cumin and coriander
- Turmeric and paprika
- Fresh cilantro for garnish
- Cooked rice for serving

Instructions:
1. In a pot, sauté diced eggplant until softened.
2. Add chickpeas, coconut milk, and spices.
3. Simmer until flavors meld and the curry thickens.
4. Garnish with fresh cilantro and serve over cooked rice.

9. Turkey and Vegetable Stir-Fry

Ingredients:
- Ground turkey
- Mixed vegetables (bell peppers, zucchini, carrots)
- Gluten-free soy sauce
- Ginger and garlic (infused oil to avoid FODMAPs)
- Green onions (green parts only)
- Sesame oil
- Cooked rice or quinoa for serving

Instructions:
1. Brown ground turkey in a pan with ginger and garlic-infused oil.
2. Add mixed vegetables and stir-fry until crisp-tender.
3. Season with gluten-free soy sauce and sesame oil.
4. Toss in green onion tops.
5. Serve over cooked rice or quinoa.

10. Nutty Energy Bites

Ingredients:
- Almond flour
- Peanut butter (with no added high FODMAP ingredients)
- Maple syrup
- Dark chocolate chips
- Chia seeds
- Vanilla extract

Instructions:
1. Mix almond flour, peanut butter, maple syrup, dark chocolate chips, chia seeds, and vanilla extract in a bowl.
2. Form small bites and refrigerate until firm.

11. Cucumber and Hummus Stacks

Ingredients:
- Cucumber, sliced
- Hummus (made with low FODMAP ingredients)
- Cherry tomatoes, halved
- Fresh basil leaves
- Olive oil drizzle
- Salt and pepper to taste

Instructions:
1. Arrange cucumber slices on a plate.
2. Spread hummus on each cucumber slice.
3. Top with cherry tomato halves and fresh basil leaves.
4. Drizzle with olive oil and season with salt and pepper.

12. Roasted Red Pepper and Feta Dip

Ingredients:
- Roasted red peppers (jarred or homemade)
- Feta cheese (without high FODMAP ingredients)
- Olive oil
- Lemon juice
- Garlic-infused oil
- Fresh parsley for garnish
- Gluten-free crackers or vegetable sticks for dipping

Instructions:
1. Blend roasted red peppers, feta cheese, olive oil, lemon juice, and garlic-infused oil until smooth.

2. Transfer to a serving bowl and garnish with fresh parsley.
3. Serve with gluten-free crackers or vegetable sticks.

13. Nutty Quinoa Breakfast Bowl

Ingredients:
- Cooked quinoa
- Sliced strawberries
- Almond butter
- Chopped walnuts
- Chia seeds
- Lactose-free yogurt
- Maple syrup (optional)

Instructions:
1. Mix cooked quinoa with sliced strawberries, almond butter, chopped walnuts, and chia seeds.
2. Top with a dollop of lactose-free yogurt.
3. Optional: Drizzle with maple syrup for sweetness.
4. Stir well and enjoy this nutty quinoa breakfast bowl.

14. Cinnamon French Toast with Blueberries

Ingredients:
- Gluten-free bread slices
- Eggs
- Lactose-free milk
- Ground cinnamon
- Blueberries
- Maple syrup (optional)

Instructions:
1. Whisk eggs, lactose-free milk, and ground cinnamon in a bowl.
2. Dip each bread slice into the egg mixture, coating both sides.
3. Cook on a griddle until golden brown.

4. Top with fresh blueberries and optional maple syrup.

15. Spinach and Feta Frittata

Ingredients:
- Eggs
- Spinach, chopped
- Feta cheese (without high FODMAP ingredients)
- Cherry tomatoes, halved
- Olive oil
- Salt and pepper to taste

Instructions:
1. Preheat the oven to 375°F (190°C).
2. Whisk eggs in a bowl and season with salt and pepper.
3. In an oven-safe skillet, sauté spinach until wilted.
4. Pour whisked eggs over spinach and add feta and cherry tomatoes.
5. Bake until the frittata is set and golden brown.

16. Raspberry Coconut Chia Pudding

Ingredients:
- Chia seeds
- Coconut milk
- Raspberries
- Shredded coconut
- Maple syrup (optional)

Instructions:
1. Mix chia seeds with coconut milk in a bowl.
2. Refrigerate for a few hours or overnight until a pudding consistency is reached.
3. Top with fresh raspberries, shredded coconut, and optional maple syrup.

17. Smoked Salmon and Avocado Toast

Ingredients:
- Gluten-free toast
- Smoked salmon
- Avocado, sliced
- Fresh dill
- Lemon juice
- Capers (optional)

Instructions:
1. Toast gluten-free bread slices.
2. Top with smoked salmon, sliced avocado, and fresh dill.
3. Drizzle with lemon juice and add capers if desired.

18. Banana Almond Butter Smoothie

Ingredients:
- Bananas
- Almond butter
- Lactose-free yogurt
- Almond milk
- Ice cubes

Instructions:
1. Blend bananas, almond butter, lactose-free yogurt, almond milk, and ice cubes until smooth.
2. Pour into a glass and enjoy this creamy banana almond butter smoothie.

19. Turkey and Spinach Breakfast Casserole

Ingredients:
- Ground turkey
- Fresh spinach
- Eggs

- Lactose-free milk
- Dijon mustard
- Nutmeg
- Salt and pepper to taste

Instructions:
1. Brown ground turkey in a pan.
2. In a bowl, whisk together eggs, lactose-free milk, Dijon mustard, nutmeg, salt, and pepper.
3. Mix in fresh spinach and cooked turkey.
4. Pour into a baking dish and bake until set.

20. Raspberry Almond Flour Muffins

Ingredients:
- Almond flour
- Eggs
- Raspberries
- Maple syrup
- Vanilla extract
- Baking powder

Instructions:
1. Mix almond flour, eggs, raspberries, maple syrup, vanilla extract, and baking powder in a bowl.
2. Spoon into muffin cups and bake until golden brown.

21. Cheddar and Chive Frittata Cups

Ingredients:
- Eggs
- Lactose-free cheddar cheese, grated
- Chives, chopped
- Salt and pepper to taste

Instructions:
1. Preheat the oven to 375°F (190°C).
2. Whisk eggs and mix in grated cheddar, chopped chives, salt, and pepper.
3. Pour into greased muffin cups and bake until set.

22. Raspberry Coconut Flour Pancakes

Ingredients:
- Coconut flour
- Eggs
- Raspberries
- Lactose-free milk
- Maple syrup

Instructions:
1. Mix coconut flour, eggs, raspberries, lactose-free milk, and maple syrup in a bowl.
2. Cook on a griddle until golden brown.

23. Cucumber and Smoked Salmon Roll-Ups

Ingredients:
- Cucumber, thinly sliced lengthwise
- Smoked salmon
- Lactose-free cream cheese
- Fresh dill

Instructions:
1. Lay out cucumber slices.
2. Spread a thin layer of lactose-free cream cheese on each slice.
3. Top with smoked salmon and fresh dill, then roll up.

24. Kiwi and Pineapple Tropical Smoothie

Ingredients:
- Kiwi, peeled and sliced
- Pineapple chunks
- Lactose-free yogurt
- Coconut water
- Ice cubes

Instructions:
1. Blend kiwi, pineapple, lactose-free yogurt, coconut water, and ice cubes until smooth.
2. Pour into a glass and enjoy this refreshing tropical smoothie.

25. Tomato and Basil Egg Muffins

Ingredients:
- Eggs
- Cherry tomatoes, halved
- Fresh basil, chopped
- Olive oil
- Salt and pepper to taste

Instructions:
1. Preheat the oven to 375°F (190°C).
2. Whisk eggs and mix in cherry tomatoes, fresh basil, olive oil, salt, and pepper.
3. Pour into greased muffin cups and bake until set.

26. Mixed Berry Coconut Chia Parfait

Ingredients:
- Mixed berries (strawberries, blueberries, raspberries)
- Chia seeds
- Coconut milk

- Maple syrup (optional)
- Shredded coconut for topping

Instructions:
1. Mix chia seeds with coconut milk and refrigerate until a pudding consistency is reached.
2. Layer chia pudding with mixed berries in a glass.
3. Optional: Drizzle with maple syrup and top with shredded coconut.

27. Apple Cinnamon Quinoa Porridge

Ingredients:
- Cooked quinoa
- Apple, diced
- Cinnamon
- Lactose-free milk
- Maple syrup (optional)
- Walnuts for topping

Instructions:
1. Mix cooked quinoa with diced apples, cinnamon, lactose-free milk, and optional maple syrup.
2. Heat until warmed through.
3. Top with walnuts and serve this cozy apple cinnamon quinoa porridge.

28. Lactose-Free Yogurt and Berry Parfait

Ingredients:
- Lactose-free yogurt
- Mixed berries (strawberries, blueberries, raspberries)
- Gluten-free granola
- Maple syrup (optional)

Instructions:
1. Layer lactose-free yogurt with mixed berries and gluten-free granola in a glass.
2. Optional: Drizzle with maple syrup for sweetness.
3. Repeat the layers and enjoy this delightful yogurt and berry parfait.

29. Dark Chocolate Almond Butter Overnight Oats

Ingredients:
- Rolled oats
- Lactose-free milk
- Almond butter
- Dark chocolate chips
- Maple syrup (optional)

Instructions:
1. Mix rolled oats with lactose-free milk, almond butter, dark chocolate chips, and optional maple syrup.
2. Refrigerate overnight.
3. Stir well before serving these indulgent dark chocolate almond butter overnight oats.

30. Almond Flour Banana Blueberry Muffins

Ingredients:
- Almond flour
- Ripe bananas, mashed
- Blueberries
- Eggs
- Maple syrup
- Baking powder

Instructions:
1. Mix almond flour, mashed bananas, blueberries, eggs, maple syrup, and baking powder in a bowl.

2. Spoon into muffin cups and bake until golden brown.

Chapter 3: Lunch

31. Grilled Chicken and Quinoa Salad

Ingredients:
- Grilled chicken breast, sliced
- Cooked quinoa
- Mixed salad greens (lettuce, spinach, arugula)
- Cherry tomatoes, halved
- Cucumber, sliced
- Olive oil
- Lemon juice
- Dijon mustard
- Salt and pepper to taste

Instructions:
1. In a large bowl, combine grilled chicken, cooked quinoa, salad greens, cherry tomatoes, and cucumber.
2. In a small bowl, whisk together olive oil, lemon juice, Dijon mustard, salt, and pepper to make the dressing.
3. Drizzle the dressing over the salad and toss gently.
4. Serve this refreshing grilled chicken and quinoa salad.

32. Low FODMAP Turkey and Cranberry Wrap

Ingredients:
- Gluten-free tortilla
- Sliced turkey breast
- Lactose-free Swiss cheese
- Spinach leaves
- Cranberry sauce (without high FODMAP ingredients)
- Mayonnaise (optional)
- Salt and pepper to taste

Instructions:
1. Lay out a gluten-free tortilla.
2. Layer sliced turkey, lactose-free Swiss cheese, and spinach leaves.
3. Add a spoonful of cranberry sauce and mayonnaise if desired.
4. Season with salt and pepper.
5. Roll up the tortilla and slice into halves or thirds.
6. This low FODMAP turkey and cranberry wrap is ready to be enjoyed.

33. Quinoa and Roasted Vegetable Buddha Bowl

Ingredients:
- Cooked quinoa
- Zucchini, sliced
- Bell peppers, sliced
- Carrots, julienned
- Olive oil
- Cumin and paprika for seasoning
- Fresh cilantro for garnish
- Optional: Grilled chicken or tofu for added protein

Instructions:
1. Toss sliced vegetables in olive oil and season with cumin and paprika.
2. Roast the vegetables until they are tender and slightly caramelized.
3. Assemble the Buddha bowl by placing a serving of quinoa in a bowl.
4. Top with roasted vegetables and your choice of protein.
5. Garnish with fresh cilantro and serve.

34. Zucchini Noodles with Pesto and Cherry Tomatoes

Ingredients:
- Zucchini, spiralized into noodles
- Cherry tomatoes, halved
- Pesto sauce (made with basil, pine nuts, Parmesan, olive oil)
- Salt and pepper to taste
- Optional: Grated Parmesan for topping

Instructions:
1. Spiralize zucchini into noodle shapes.
2. In a pan, sauté zucchini noodles until just tender.
3. Mix in pesto sauce and cherry tomatoes.
4. Season with salt and pepper to taste.
5. Optional: Top with grated Parmesan before serving.

35. Baked Salmon with Dill and Lemon

Ingredients:
- Salmon fillets
- Fresh dill, chopped
- Lemon slices
- Olive oil
- Salt and pepper to taste

Instructions:
1. Preheat the oven to 375°F (190°C).
2. Place salmon fillets on a baking sheet.
3. Drizzle with olive oil and sprinkle with fresh dill, salt, and pepper.
4. Top each fillet with lemon slices.
5. Bake for 15-20 minutes or until the salmon flakes easily with a fork.

36. Eggplant and Chickpea Curry

Ingredients:
- Eggplant, diced
- Canned chickpeas, drained and rinsed
- Coconut milk
- Curry powder
- Cumin and coriander
- Turmeric and paprika
- Fresh cilantro for garnish
- Cooked rice for serving

Instructions:
1. In a pot, sauté diced eggplant until softened.
2. Add chickpeas, coconut milk, and spices.
3. Simmer until flavors meld and the curry thickens.
4. Garnish with fresh cilantro and serve over cooked rice.

37. Turkey and Vegetable Stir-Fry

Ingredients:
- Ground turkey
- Mixed vegetables (bell peppers, zucchini, carrots)
- Gluten-free soy sauce
- Ginger and garlic (infused oil to avoid FODMAPs)
- Green onions (green parts only)
- Sesame oil
- Cooked rice or quinoa for serving

Instructions:
1. Brown ground turkey in a pan with ginger and garlic-infused oil.
2. Add mixed vegetables and stir-fry until crisp-tender.
3. Season with gluten-free soy sauce and sesame oil.
4. Toss in green onion tops.
5. Serve over cooked rice or quinoa.

38. Lemon Herb Grilled Chicken Salad

Ingredients:
- Grilled chicken breast, sliced
- Mixed salad greens (lettuce, spinach, arugula)
- Cherry tomatoes, halved
- Cucumber, sliced
- Olive oil
- Lemon juice
- Dijon mustard
- Salt and pepper to taste

Instructions:
1. In a large bowl, combine grilled chicken, salad greens, cherry tomatoes, and cucumber.
2. In a small bowl, whisk together olive oil, lemon juice, Dijon mustard, salt, and pepper to make the dressing.
3. Drizzle the dressing over the salad and toss gently.
4. This lemon herb grilled chicken salad is a delightful and light lunch option.

39. Quinoa and Roasted Vegetable Buddha Bowl

Ingredients:
- Cooked quinoa
- Zucchini, sliced
- Bell peppers, sliced
- Carrots, julienned
- Olive oil
- Cumin and paprika for seasoning
- Fresh cilantro for garnish
- Optional: Grilled chicken or tofu for added protein

Instructions:
1. Toss sliced vegetables in olive oil and season with cumin and paprika.
2. Roast the vegetables until they are tender and slightly caramelized.
3. Assemble the Buddha bowl by placing a serving of quinoa in a bowl.
4. Top with roasted vegetables and your choice of protein.
5. Garnish with fresh cilantro and serve.

40. Zucchini Noodles with Pesto and Cherry Tomatoes

Ingredients:
- Zucchini, spiralized into noodles
- Cherry tomatoes, halved
- Pesto sauce (made with basil, pine nuts, Parmesan, olive oil)

- Salt and pepper to taste
- Optional: Grated Parmesan for topping

Instructions:
1. Spiralize zucchini into noodle shapes.
2. In a pan, sauté zucchini noodles until just tender.
3. Mix in pesto sauce and cherry tomatoes.
4. Season with salt and pepper to taste.
5. Optional: Top with grated Parmesan before serving.

41. Satisfying Eggplant and Chickpea Curry

Ingredients:
- Eggplant, diced
- Canned chickpeas, drained and rinsed
- Coconut milk
- Curry powder
- Cumin and coriander
- Turmeric and paprika
- Fresh cilantro for garnish
- Cooked rice for serving

Instructions:
1. In a pot, sauté diced eggplant until softened.
2. Add chickpeas, coconut milk, and spices.
3. Simmer until flavors meld and the curry thickens.
4. Garnish with fresh cilantro and serve over cooked rice.

42. Turkey and Vegetable Stir-Fry

Ingredients:
- Ground turkey
- Mixed vegetables (bell peppers, zucchini, carrots)
- Gluten-free soy sauce
- Ginger and garlic (infused oil to avoid FODMAPs)

- Green onions (green parts only)
- Sesame oil
- Cooked rice or quinoa for serving

Instructions:
1. Brown ground turkey in a pan with ginger and garlic-infused oil.
2. Add mixed vegetables and stir-fry until crisp-tender.
3. Season with gluten-free soy sauce and sesame oil.
4. Toss in green onion tops.
5. Serve over cooked rice or quinoa.

43. Tomato Basil Chicken Salad

Ingredients:
- Grilled chicken breast, sliced
- Mixed salad greens (lettuce, spinach, arugula)
- Cherry tomatoes, halved
- Fresh basil leaves, torn
- Balsamic vinaigrette (made with low FODMAP ingredients)
- Salt and pepper to taste

Instructions:
1. In a large bowl, combine grilled chicken, salad greens, cherry tomatoes, and torn basil leaves.
2. Drizzle with balsamic vinaigrette and toss gently.
3. Season with salt and pepper to taste.
4. This tomato basil chicken salad is a light and flavorful lunch option.

44. Quinoa Stuffed Bell Peppers

Ingredients:
- Bell peppers, halved and cleaned
- Cooked quinoa
- Ground turkey
- Tomato sauce (made with low FODMAP ingredients)

- Zucchini, diced
- Olive oil
- Italian seasoning
- Salt and pepper to taste

Instructions:
1. Preheat the oven to 375°F (190°C).
2. In a skillet, brown ground turkey with diced zucchini in olive oil.
3. Mix cooked quinoa, browned turkey, tomato sauce, Italian seasoning, salt, and pepper in a bowl.
4. Stuff bell peppers with the quinoa mixture.
5. Bake until the peppers are tender.

45. Caprese Salad with Balsamic Glaze

Ingredients:
- Fresh mozzarella, sliced
- Cherry tomatoes, halved
- Fresh basil leaves
- Balsamic glaze (made with low FODMAP ingredients)
- Olive oil
- Salt and pepper to taste

Instructions:
1. Arrange slices of fresh mozzarella and cherry tomatoes on a plate.
2. Tuck fresh basil leaves between the cheese and tomatoes.
3. Drizzle with balsamic glaze and olive oil.
4. Season with salt and pepper to taste.

46. Lemony Shrimp and Spinach Risotto

Ingredients:
- Arborio rice
- Shrimp, peeled and deveined
- Baby spinach

- Chicken or vegetable broth (low FODMAP)
- Lemon zest
- Parmesan cheese (optional)
- Olive oil
- Salt and pepper to taste

Instructions:
1. In a pan, sauté shrimp in olive oil until cooked.
2. Add Arborio rice and cook until lightly toasted.
3. Gradually add low FODMAP broth, stirring until absorbed.
4. Stir in baby spinach and lemon zest.
5. Optional: Add Parmesan cheese for extra creaminess.
6. Season with salt and pepper to taste.

47. Turkey and Cranberry Quinoa Bowl

Ingredients:
- Cooked quinoa
- Ground turkey
- Cranberry sauce (without high FODMAP ingredients)
- Green beans, blanched
- Almonds, sliced
- Olive oil
- Salt and pepper to taste

Instructions:
1. In a skillet, brown ground turkey in olive oil.
2. Mix cooked quinoa, browned turkey, cranberry sauce, blanched green beans, and sliced almonds in a bowl.
3. Season with salt and pepper to taste.
4. This turkey and cranberry quinoa bowl is a satisfying and balanced lunch.

48. Spinach and Feta Stuffed Chicken Breast

Ingredients:
- Boneless, skinless chicken breasts
- Fresh spinach leaves
- Feta cheese (low FODMAP)
- Olive oil
- Lemon juice
- Garlic-infused oil
- Salt and pepper to taste

Instructions:
1. Preheat your oven to 375°F (190°C).
2. Butterfly the chicken breasts by slicing them horizontally without cutting all the way through.
3. Lay the chicken breasts flat and season with salt and pepper.
4. In a skillet, sauté fresh spinach in a bit of olive oil until wilted. Drain excess liquid.
5. Stuff each chicken breast with a generous amount of fresh spinach and crumbled feta.
6. Drizzle with olive oil, lemon juice, and a touch of garlic-infused oil.
7. Carefully close the chicken breasts and secure with toothpicks.
8. Place the stuffed chicken breasts on a baking sheet and bake for approximately 25-30 minutes or until the chicken is cooked through.
9. Remove toothpicks before serving.

49. Chicken and Vegetable Skewers

Ingredients:
- Chicken breast, cut into cubes
- Zucchini, sliced
- Cherry tomatoes
- Red bell pepper, diced
- Olive oil
- Lemon juice

- Dried oregano
- Salt and pepper to taste

Instructions:
1. Thread chicken cubes, zucchini slices, cherry tomatoes, and red bell pepper onto skewers.
2. Mix olive oil, lemon juice, dried oregano, salt, and pepper to create a marinade.
3. Brush the skewers with the marinade and grill until chicken is cooked through.

50. Shrimp and Quinoa Stir-Fry

Ingredients:
- Shrimp, peeled and deveined
- Cooked quinoa
- Bok choy, chopped
- Carrots, julienned
- Gluten-free soy sauce
- Sesame oil
- Ginger (infused oil to avoid FODMAPs)
- Green onions (green parts only)
- Sesame seeds for garnish

Instructions:
1. Stir-fry shrimp, bok choy, and carrots in sesame oil and ginger-infused oil.
2. Add cooked quinoa and gluten-free soy sauce.
3. Toss in green onion tops and garnish with sesame seeds.

51. Mediterranean Chicken Wrap

Ingredients:
- Grilled chicken strips
- Gluten-free wrap

- Romaine lettuce leaves
- Kalamata olives, sliced
- Cucumber, diced
- Cherry tomatoes, halved
- Feta cheese (without high FODMAP ingredients)
- Greek dressing (made with low FODMAP ingredients)

Instructions:
1. Lay out a gluten-free wrap.
2. Layer grilled chicken strips, romaine lettuce, olives, cucumber, cherry tomatoes, and crumbled feta.
3. Drizzle with Greek dressing.
4. Roll up the wrap and enjoy this Mediterranean-inspired delight.

52. Quinoa and Roasted Butternut Squash Salad

Ingredients:
- Cooked quinoa
- Roasted butternut squash cubes
- Baby spinach leaves
- Pomegranate arils
- Pecans, chopped
- Olive oil
- Balsamic vinegar (made with low FODMAP ingredients)
- Maple syrup (optional)
- Salt and pepper to taste

Instructions:
1. In a large bowl, combine cooked quinoa, roasted butternut squash, baby spinach, pomegranate arils, and chopped pecans.
2. Whisk together olive oil, balsamic vinegar, maple syrup (if using), salt, and pepper to make the dressing.
3. Drizzle the dressing over the salad and toss gently.

53. Tuna and Avocado Salad

Ingredients:
- Canned tuna, drained
- Avocado, diced
- Romaine lettuce leaves
- Cherry tomatoes, halved
- Cucumber, sliced
- Olive oil
- Lemon juice
- Dijon mustard
- Salt and pepper to taste

Instructions:
1. In a bowl, mix canned tuna, diced avocado, romaine lettuce, cherry tomatoes, and cucumber.
2. In a small bowl, whisk together olive oil, lemon juice, Dijon mustard, salt, and pepper to make the dressing.
3. Drizzle the dressing over the tuna and avocado salad and toss gently.

54. Quinoa and Kale Stuffed Peppers

Ingredients:
- Bell peppers, halved and cleaned
- Cooked quinoa
- Fresh kale, chopped
- Ground turkey
- Tomato sauce (made with low FODMAP ingredients)
- Olive oil
- Italian seasoning
- Salt and pepper to taste

Instructions:
1. Preheat the oven to 375°F (190°C).
2. In a skillet, brown ground turkey in olive oil.

3. Mix cooked quinoa, fresh kale, browned turkey, tomato sauce, Italian seasoning, salt, and pepper in a bowl.
4. Stuff bell peppers with the quinoa and turkey mixture.
5. Bake until the peppers are tender.

55. Asian-Inspired Beef Lettuce Wraps

Ingredients:
- Ground beef
- Butter lettuce leaves
- Carrots, julienned
- Water chestnuts, sliced
- Green onions (green parts only)
- Ginger (infused oil to avoid FODMAPs)
- Gluten-free soy sauce
- Sesame oil
- Sesame seeds for garnish

Instructions:
1. Brown ground beef in a pan with ginger-infused oil.
2. Add julienned carrots, water chestnuts, and green onion tops.
3. Season with gluten-free soy sauce and sesame oil.
4. Spoon the mixture onto butter lettuce leaves and sprinkle with sesame seeds.

56. Caprese Quinoa Bowl

Ingredients:
- Cooked quinoa
- Cherry tomatoes, halved
- Fresh mozzarella, diced
- Fresh basil leaves, torn
- Balsamic glaze (made with low FODMAP ingredients)
- Olive oil
- Salt and pepper to taste

Instructions:
1. In a bowl, combine cooked quinoa, cherry tomatoes, fresh mozzarella, and torn basil leaves.
2. Drizzle with balsamic glaze and olive oil.
3. Season with salt and pepper to taste.

57. Spaghetti Squash with Pesto and Cherry Tomatoes

Ingredients:
- Spaghetti squash, cooked and shredded
- Pesto sauce (made with basil, pine nuts, Parmesan, olive oil)
- Cherry tomatoes, halved
- Olive oil
- Salt and pepper to taste
- Optional: Grated Parmesan for topping

Instructions:
1. In a bowl, mix shredded spaghetti squash with pesto sauce and cherry tomatoes.
2. Drizzle with olive oil and season with salt and pepper.
3. Optional: Top with grated Parmesan before serving.

58. Turkey and Spinach Stuffed Portobello Mushrooms

Ingredients:
- Portobello mushrooms, cleaned
- Ground turkey
- Fresh spinach
- Olive oil
- Garlic-infused oil
- Italian seasoning
- Salt and pepper to taste

Instructions:
1. Preheat the oven to 375°F (190°C).

2. In a skillet, brown ground turkey in olive oil and garlic-infused oil.
3. Add fresh spinach and cook until wilted.
4. Season with Italian seasoning, salt, and pepper.
5. Stuff portobello mushrooms with the turkey and spinach mixture.
6. Bake until mushrooms are tender.

59. Chicken and Vegetable Stir-Fry with Pineapple

Ingredients:
- Chicken breast, sliced
- Mixed vegetables (bell peppers, broccoli, carrots)
- Pineapple chunks
- Gluten-free soy sauce
- Ginger (infused oil to avoid FODMAPs)
- Sesame oil
- Green onions (green parts only)
- Cooked rice for serving

Instructions
1. Stir-fry chicken, mixed vegetables, and pineapple in ginger-infused oil and sesame oil.
2. Season with gluten-free soy sauce.
3. Toss in green onion tops.
4. Serve over cooked rice.

60. Spinach and Tomato Omelette

Ingredients:
- Eggs
- Fresh spinach
- Cherry tomatoes, halved
- Lactose-free feta cheese
- Olive oil
- Salt and pepper to taste

Instructions:
1. In a bowl, whisk eggs and season with salt and pepper.
2. In a pan, sauté fresh spinach until wilted.
3. Pour whisked eggs over the spinach.
4. Add halved cherry tomatoes and crumbled lactose-free feta.
5. Cook until the omelette is set.

Chapter 4: Dinners

61. Grilled Lemon Garlic Shrimp Skewers

Ingredients:
- Shrimp, peeled and deveined
- Lemon juice
- Garlic-infused oil
- Fresh parsley, chopped
- Salt and pepper to taste

Instructions:
1. In a bowl, mix shrimp with lemon juice, garlic-infused oil, chopped parsley, salt, and pepper.
2. Thread shrimp onto skewers and grill until cooked.
3. Serve these flavorful grilled lemon garlic shrimp skewers.

62. Baked Chicken Parmesan

Ingredients:
- Chicken breasts, boneless and skinless
- Gluten-free breadcrumbs
- Parmesan cheese (low FODMAP)
- Tomato sauce (made with low FODMAP ingredients)
- Mozzarella cheese, shredded
- Olive oil
- Fresh basil leaves for garnish

Instructions:
1. Preheat the oven to 375°F (190°C).
2. Coat chicken breasts with a mixture of gluten-free breadcrumbs and Parmesan cheese.
3. Place the coated chicken breasts in a baking dish and top with tomato sauce and shredded mozzarella.

4. Drizzle with olive oil and bake until the chicken is cooked through and the cheese is melted and bubbly.
5. Garnish with fresh basil leaves before serving.

63. Lemon Herb Baked Cod

Ingredients:
- Cod fillets
- Lemon zest
- Fresh dill, chopped
- Olive oil
- Salt and pepper to taste

Instructions:
1. Preheat the oven to 375°F (190°C).
2. Place cod fillets on a baking sheet.
3. Sprinkle with lemon zest, chopped fresh dill, olive oil, salt, and pepper.
4. Bake until the cod is flaky and cooked through.
5. Enjoy this light and flavorful lemon herb baked cod.

64. Quinoa-Stuffed Bell Peppers

Ingredients:
- Bell peppers, halved and cleaned
- Cooked quinoa
- Ground turkey
- Tomato sauce (made with low FODMAP ingredients)
- Zucchini, diced
- Olive oil
- Italian seasoning
- Salt and pepper to taste

Instructions:
1. Preheat the oven to 375°F (190°C).
2. In a skillet, brown ground turkey with diced zucchini in olive oil.

3. Mix cooked quinoa, browned turkey, tomato sauce, Italian seasoning, salt, and pepper in a bowl.
4. Stuff bell peppers with the quinoa mixture.
5. Bake until the peppers are tender.

65. Chicken and Vegetable Stir-Fry with Pineapple

Ingredients:
- Chicken breast, sliced
- Mixed vegetables (bell peppers, broccoli, carrots)
- Pineapple chunks
- Gluten-free soy sauce
- Ginger (infused oil to avoid FODMAPs)
- Sesame oil
- Green onions (green parts only)
- Cooked rice for serving

Instructions:
1. Stir-fry chicken, mixed vegetables, and pineapple in ginger-infused oil and sesame oil.
2. Season with gluten-free soy sauce.
3. Toss in green onion tops.
4. Serve over cooked rice.

66. Spaghetti Squash with Pesto and Cherry Tomatoes

Ingredients:
- Spaghetti squash, cooked and shredded
- Pesto sauce (made with basil, pine nuts, Parmesan, olive oil)
- Cherry tomatoes, halved
- Olive oil
- Salt and pepper to taste
- Optional: Grated Parmesan for topping

Instructions:
1. In a bowl, mix shredded spaghetti squash with pesto sauce and cherry tomatoes.
2. Drizzle with olive oil and season with salt and pepper.
3. Optional: Top with grated Parmesan before serving.

67. Turkey and Spinach Stuffed Portobello Mushrooms

Ingredients:
- Portobello mushrooms, cleaned
- Ground turkey
- Fresh spinach
- Olive oil
- Garlic-infused oil
- Italian seasoning
- Salt and pepper to taste

Instructions:
1. Preheat the oven to 375°F (190°C).
2. In a skillet, brown ground turkey in olive oil and garlic-infused oil.
3. Add fresh spinach and cook until wilted.
4. Season with Italian seasoning, salt, and pepper.
5. Stuff portobello mushrooms with the turkey and spinach mixture.
6. Bake until mushrooms are tender.

68. Asian-Inspired Beef Lettuce Wraps

Ingredients:
- Ground beef
- Butter lettuce leaves
- Carrots, julienned
- Water chestnuts, sliced
- Green onions (green parts only)
- Ginger (infused oil to avoid FODMAPs)
- Gluten-free soy sauce

- Sesame oil
- Sesame seeds for garnish

Instructions:
1. Brown ground beef in a pan with ginger-infused oil.
2. Add julienned carrots, water chestnuts, and green onion tops.
3. Season with gluten-free soy sauce and sesame oil.
4. Spoon the mixture onto butter lettuce leaves and sprinkle with sesame seeds.

69. Caprese Quinoa Bowl

Ingredients:
- Cooked quinoa
- Cherry tomatoes, halved
- Fresh mozzarella, diced
- Fresh basil leaves, torn
- Balsamic glaze (made with low FODMAP ingredients)
- Olive oil
- Salt and pepper to taste

Instructions:
1. In a bowl, combine cooked quinoa, cherry tomatoes, fresh mozzarella, and torn basil leaves.
2. Drizzle with balsamic glaze and olive oil.
3. Season with salt and pepper to taste.

70. Spiced Turkey and Butternut Squash Skillet

Ingredients:
- Ground turkey
- Butternut squash, diced
- Green beans, trimmed
- Cumin and paprika
- Olive oil

- Garlic-infused oil
- Salt and pepper to taste

Instructions:
1. In a skillet, brown ground turkey in olive oil and garlic-infused oil.
2. Add diced butternut squash and green beans.
3. Season with cumin, paprika, salt, and pepper.
4. Cook until the vegetables are tender and the turkey is cooked through.

71. Lemon Rosemary Roasted Chicken Thighs

Ingredients:
- Chicken thighs, bone-in and skin-on
- Lemon zest
- Fresh rosemary, chopped
- Olive oil
- Salt and pepper to taste

Instructions:
1. Preheat the oven to 400°F (200°C).
2. Place chicken thighs on a baking sheet.
3. Sprinkle with lemon zest, chopped fresh rosemary, olive oil, salt, and pepper.
4. Roast until the chicken is golden brown and cooked through.

72. Shrimp and Vegetable Stir-Fry

Ingredients:
- Shrimp, peeled and deveined
- Mixed vegetables (bell peppers, broccoli, carrots)
- Gluten-free soy sauce
- Ginger (infused oil to avoid FODMAPs)
- Sesame oil
- Green onions (green parts only)
- Cooked rice for serving

Instructions:
1. Stir-fry shrimp and mixed vegetables in ginger-infused oil and sesame oil.
2. Season with gluten-free soy sauce.
3. Toss in green onion tops.
4. Serve over cooked rice.

73. Zucchini and Turkey Meatballs

Ingredients:
- Ground turkey
- Zucchini, grated and excess moisture squeezed out
- Gluten-free breadcrumbs
- Parmesan cheese (low FODMAP)
- Tomato sauce (made with low FODMAP ingredients)
- Olive oil
- Fresh basil leaves for garnish

Instructions:
1. Preheat the oven to 375°F (190°C).
2. In a bowl, mix ground turkey, grated zucchini, gluten-free breadcrumbs, and Parmesan cheese.
3. Form the mixture into meatballs and place them on a baking sheet.
4. Bake until the meatballs are cooked through.
5. Heat tomato sauce in a pan, add the meatballs, and simmer until warmed.
6. Garnish with fresh basil leaves before serving.

74. Quinoa and Vegetable Stuffed Peppers

Ingredients:
- Bell peppers, halved and cleaned
- Cooked quinoa
- Mixed vegetables (zucchini, cherry tomatoes, spinach)
- Olive oil
- Lemon juice

- Dried oregano
- Salt and pepper to taste

Instructions:
1. Preheat the oven to 375°F (190°C).
2. In a bowl, combine cooked quinoa, mixed vegetables, olive oil, lemon juice, dried oregano, salt, and pepper.
3. Stuff bell peppers with the quinoa and vegetable mixture.
4. Bake until the peppers are tender.

75. Teriyaki Chicken Skewers

Ingredients:
- Chicken breast, cut into cubes
- Gluten-free teriyaki sauce
- Pineapple chunks
- Green bell pepper, diced
- Olive oil
- Sesame seeds for garnish

Instructions:
1. Marinate chicken cubes in gluten-free teriyaki sauce.
2. Thread marinated chicken, pineapple chunks, and diced green bell pepper onto skewers.
3. Grill until the chicken is cooked through.
4. Drizzle with olive oil and sprinkle with sesame seeds before serving.

76. Mediterranean Quinoa Salad

Ingredients:
- Cooked quinoa
- Cherry tomatoes, halved
- Cucumber, diced
- Kalamata olives, sliced
- Feta cheese (low FODMAP)

- Olive oil
- Lemon juice
- Fresh oregano leaves for garnish

Instructions:
1. In a bowl, combine cooked quinoa, cherry tomatoes, diced cucumber, sliced Kalamata olives, and crumbled feta.
2. Drizzle with olive oil and lemon juice.
3. Toss gently and garnish with fresh oregano leaves.

77. Thai-Inspired Ground Turkey Lettuce Wraps

Ingredients:
- Ground turkey
- Butter lettuce leaves
- Carrots, julienned
- Red bell pepper, diced
- Mint leaves
- Gluten-free hoisin sauce
- Lime wedges for serving

Instructions:
1. Brown ground turkey in a pan.
2. Add julienned carrots, diced red bell pepper, and gluten-free hoisin sauce.
3. Spoon the mixture onto butter lettuce leaves.
4. Top with fresh mint leaves.
5. Serve with lime wedges for squeezing.

78. Eggplant Parmesan

Ingredients:
- Eggplant, sliced
- Gluten-free breadcrumbs
- Parmesan cheese (low FODMAP)

- Tomato sauce (made with low FODMAP ingredients)
- Mozzarella cheese, shredded
- Olive oil
- Fresh basil leaves for garnish

Instructions:
1. Preheat the oven to 375°F (190°C).
2. Coat eggplant slices with a mixture of gluten-free breadcrumbs and Parmesan cheese.
3. Arrange the coated eggplant slices in a baking dish.
4. Top with tomato sauce and shredded mozzarella.
5. Drizzle with olive oil and bake until the eggplant is tender and the cheese is bubbly.
6. Garnish with fresh basil leaves before serving.

79. Lemon Dill Baked Salmon

Ingredients:
- Salmon fillets
- Lemon slices
- Fresh dill, chopped
- Olive oil
- Salt and pepper to taste

Instructions:
1. Preheat the oven to 375°F (190°C).
2. Place salmon

fillets on a baking sheet.
3. Top with lemon slices, chopped fresh dill, olive oil, salt, and pepper.
4. Bake until the salmon is flaky and cooked through.

80. Cumin-Spiced Beef and Vegetable Skewers

Ingredients:
- Beef sirloin, cut into cubes
- Zucchini, sliced
- Cherry tomatoes
- Red onion, diced
- Cumin and paprika
- Olive oil
- Salt and pepper to taste

Instructions:
1. In a bowl, mix beef cubes, sliced zucchini, cherry tomatoes, diced red onion, cumin, paprika, olive oil, salt, and pepper.
2. Thread the mixture onto skewers and grill until the beef is cooked to your liking.
3. Serve these flavorful cumin-spiced beef and vegetable skewers.

Chapter 5: Snacks and Quick Bites

81. Nutty Energy Bites

Ingredients:
- Almond butter (low FODMAP)
- Rolled oats
- Chia seeds
- Maple syrup (low FODMAP)
- Vanilla extract
- Dark chocolate chips (low FODMAP)
- Shredded coconut (optional)

Instructions:
1. In a bowl, mix almond butter, rolled oats, chia seeds, maple syrup, and vanilla extract until well combined.
2. Fold in dark chocolate chips.
3. Roll the mixture into bite-sized balls.
4. Optional: Roll the energy bites in shredded coconut.
5. Chill in the refrigerator before serving.

82. Cucumber and Hummus Stacks

Ingredients:
- Cucumber, sliced
- Hummus (low FODMAP)
- Cherry tomatoes, halved
- Fresh basil leaves
- Olive oil
- Salt and pepper to taste

Instructions:
1. Place a cucumber slice on a serving platter.
2. Spread a layer of hummus on top.
3. Add a cherry tomato half and a fresh basil leaf.

4. Drizzle with olive oil and season with salt and pepper.
5. Repeat to create cucumber and hummus stacks.

83. Roasted Red Pepper and Feta Dip

Ingredients:
- Roasted red peppers (from a jar, drained)
- Feta cheese (low FODMAP)
- Olive oil
- Lemon juice
- Fresh parsley, chopped
- Gluten-free crackers or vegetable sticks for dipping

Instructions:
1. In a food processor, combine roasted red peppers, feta cheese, olive oil, and lemon juice.
2. Blend until smooth and creamy.
3. Transfer the dip to a bowl and stir in chopped fresh parsley.
4. Serve with gluten-free crackers or vegetable sticks.

84. Caprese Skewers

Ingredients:
- Cherry tomatoes
- Fresh mozzarella balls (low FODMAP)
- Fresh basil leaves
- Balsamic glaze (made with low FODMAP ingredients)
- Toothpicks

Instructions:
1. Thread a cherry tomato, a mozzarella ball, and a fresh basil leaf onto a toothpick.
2. Arrange the caprese skewers on a serving platter.
3. Drizzle with balsamic glaze before serving.

85. Smoked Salmon and Cucumber Bites

Ingredients:
- English cucumber, sliced
- Smoked salmon
- Lactose-free cream cheese
- Fresh dill, chopped
- Lemon zest
- Black pepper

Instructions:
1. Top each cucumber slice with a small piece of smoked salmon.
2. In a bowl, mix lactose-free cream cheese, chopped fresh dill, and lemon zest.
3. Place a dollop of the cream cheese mixture on the smoked salmon.
4. Sprinkle with black pepper before serving.

86. Olive and Herb Quinoa Crackers

Ingredients:
- Cooked quinoa
- Kalamata olives, finely chopped
- Fresh rosemary, chopped
- Olive oil
- Salt and pepper to taste

Instructions:
1. Preheat the oven to 350°F (175°C).
2. In a bowl, combine cooked quinoa, chopped Kalamata olives, chopped fresh rosemary, olive oil, salt, and pepper.
3. Spread the mixture onto a lined baking sheet and press it into a thin layer.
4. Bake until the edges are golden brown.
5. Allow to cool, then break into crackers.

87. Greek Yogurt Parfait with Berries

Ingredients:
- Lactose-free Greek yogurt
- Low FODMAP granola
- Mixed berries (strawberries, blueberries, raspberries)
- Maple syrup (low FODMAP)

Instructions:
1. In a glass or bowl, layer lactose-free Greek yogurt, low FODMAP granola, and mixed berries.
2. Repeat the layers.
3. Drizzle with maple syrup before serving.

88. Pesto and Tomato Rice Cakes

Ingredients:
- Rice cakes (check for low FODMAP ingredients)
- Basil pesto (made with low FODMAP ingredients)
- Cherry tomatoes, sliced
- Fresh basil leaves
- Salt and pepper to taste

Instructions:
1. Spread a layer of basil pesto on each rice cake.
2. Top with sliced cherry tomatoes and fresh basil leaves.
3. Season with salt and pepper before serving.

89. Lemony Almond Flour Banana Bread Bites

Ingredients:
- Almond flour banana bread (sliced into bite-sized pieces)
- Almond butter (low FODMAP)
- Sliced bananas
- Lemon zest

Instructions:
1. Spread a thin layer of almond butter on each banana bread bite.
2. Top with sliced bananas.
3. Sprinkle with lemon zest before serving.

90. Spiced Roasted Chickpeas

Ingredients:
- Canned chickpeas, drained and rinsed
- Olive oil
- Smoked paprika
- Cumin
- Garlic-infused oil
- Salt and pepper to taste

Instructions:
1. Preheat the oven to 400°F (200°C).
2. In a bowl, toss chickpeas with olive oil, smoked paprika, cumin, garlic-infused oil, salt, and pepper.
3. Spread the chickpeas on a baking sheet and roast until crispy.
4. Allow to cool before serving.

Chapter 6: Sweet Treats

91. Berry Chia Seed Pudding

Ingredients:
- Lactose-free yogurt
- Mixed berries (strawberries, blueberries, raspberries)
- Chia seeds
- Maple syrup (low FODMAP)
- Vanilla extract

Instructions:
1. In a bowl, mix lactose-free yogurt, chia seeds, maple syrup, and vanilla extract.
2. Layer the chia seed mixture with mixed berries in serving glasses.
3. Refrigerate overnight to allow the chia seeds to absorb the liquid.
4. Serve chilled.

92. Dark Chocolate Avocado Mousse

Ingredients:
- Ripe avocados
- Dark chocolate (low FODMAP), melted
- Maple syrup (low FODMAP)
- Unsweetened cocoa powder
- Vanilla extract
- Pinch of salt
- Fresh berries for garnish

Instructions:
1. In a blender, combine ripe avocados, melted dark chocolate, maple syrup, cocoa powder, vanilla extract, and a pinch of salt.
2. Blend until smooth and creamy.
3. Chill in the refrigerator.
4. Serve topped with fresh berries.

93. Almond Flour Banana Bread

Ingredients:
- Ripe bananas
- Almond flour
- Eggs
- Maple syrup (low FODMAP)
- Baking soda
- Cinnamon
- Vanilla extract
- Salt
- Chopped walnuts (optional)

Instructions:
1. Preheat the oven to 350°F (175°C) and grease a loaf pan.
2. In a bowl, mash ripe bananas.
3. Add almond flour, eggs, maple syrup, baking soda, cinnamon, vanilla extract, and salt. Mix well.
4. Fold in chopped walnuts if desired.
5. Pour the batter into the loaf pan and bake until a toothpick inserted comes out clean.
6. Allow to cool before slicing.

94. Lemon Poppy Seed Muffins

Ingredients:
- Gluten-free flour
- Poppy seeds
- Lactose-free yogurt
- Lemon zest
- Lemon juice
- Eggs
- Maple syrup (low FODMAP)
- Baking powder
- Vanilla extract

- Olive oil

Instructions:
1. Preheat the oven to 375°F (190°C) and line a muffin tin with paper liners.
2. In a bowl, whisk together gluten-free flour, poppy seeds, baking powder, and a pinch of salt.
3. In another bowl, mix lactose-free yogurt, lemon zest, lemon juice, eggs, maple syrup, vanilla extract, and olive oil.
4. Combine the wet and dry ingredients until just combined.
5. Spoon the batter into the muffin tin and bake until golden brown.
6. Allow the muffins to cool before serving.

95. Maple Cinnamon Roasted Pecans

Ingredients:
- Pecan halves
- Maple syrup (low FODMAP)
- Ground cinnamon
- Sea salt

Instructions:
1. Preheat the oven to 325°F (163°C) and line a baking sheet with parchment paper.
2. In a bowl, toss pecan halves with maple syrup, ground cinnamon, and a pinch of sea salt.
3. Spread the pecans on the baking sheet and bake until toasted.
4. Allow to cool before serving.

96. Orange and Almond Cake

Ingredients:
- Almond flour
- Oranges
- Eggs
- Maple syrup (low FODMAP)

- Baking powder
- Vanilla extract
- Olive oil
- Orange zest for garnish

Instructions:
1. Preheat the oven to 350°F (175°C) and grease a cake pan.
2. Boil whole oranges until soft, then blend them into a puree.
3. In a bowl, mix almond flour, eggs, maple syrup, baking powder, vanilla extract, olive oil, and the orange puree.
4. Pour the batter into the cake pan and bake until a toothpick inserted comes out clean.
5. Allow the cake to cool before garnishing with orange zest.

97. Coconut and Raspberry Panna Cotta

Ingredients:
- Coconut milk
- Gelatin
- Maple syrup (low FODMAP)
- Vanilla extract
- Raspberries for topping

Instructions:
1. In a saucepan, heat coconut milk until warm.
2. Sprinkle gelatin over the coconut milk and whisk until dissolved.
3. Stir in maple syrup and vanilla extract.
4. Pour the mixture into individual serving glasses.
5. Refrigerate until set.
6. Top with fresh raspberries before serving.

98. Pistachio and Raspberry Frozen Yogurt

Ingredients:
- Lactose-free yogurt

- Maple syrup (low FODMAP)
- Pistachios, chopped
- Raspberries
- Vanilla extract

Instructions:
1. In a blender, combine lactose-free yogurt, maple syrup, chopped pistachios, raspberries, and vanilla extract.
2. Blend until smooth.
3. Pour the mixture into an ice cream maker and churn according to the manufacturer's instructions.
4. Transfer to a container and freeze until firm.
5. Serve scoops of pistachio and raspberry frozen yogurt.

99. Chocolate Covered Strawberries

Ingredients:
- Strawberries
- Dark chocolate (low FODMAP), melted
- Chopped nuts (optional)

Instructions:
1. Wash and dry strawberries, leaving the stems intact.
2. Dip each strawberry into melted dark chocolate.
3. Place on a parchment-lined tray.
4. Optional: Sprinkle with chopped nuts.
5. Allow the chocolate to set before serving.

100. Vanilla Coconut Bliss Balls

Ingredients:
- Shredded coconut
- Almond flour
- Maple syrup (low FODMAP)
- Vanilla extract

- Coconut oil, melted

Instructions:
1. In a bowl, combine shredded coconut, almond flour, maple syrup, vanilla extract, and melted coconut oil.
2. Roll the mixture into small bliss balls.
3. Chill in the refrigerator before serving.

Chapter 7: 28-Day Meal Plan

-Week 1:

Day 1:
- Breakfast: Energizing Quinoa Breakfast Bowl
- Lunch: Lemon Herb Grilled Chicken Salad
- Dinner: Baked Salmon with Dill and Lemon

Day 2:
- Breakfast: Blueberry Almond Smoothie
- Lunch: Quinoa and Roasted Vegetable Buddha Bowl
- Dinner: Eggplant and Chickpea Curry

Day 3:
- Breakfast: Scrambled Tofu with Spinach and Tomatoes
- Lunch: Zucchini Noodles with Pesto and Cherry Tomatoes
- Dinner: Turkey and Vegetable Stir-Fry

Day 4:
- Breakfast: Energizing Quinoa Breakfast Bowl
- Lunch: Lemon Herb Grilled Chicken Salad
- Dinner: Baked Salmon with Dill and Lemon

Day 5:
- Breakfast: Blueberry Almond Smoothie
- Lunch: Quinoa and Roasted Vegetable Buddha Bowl
- Dinner: Eggplant and Chickpea Curry

Day 6:
- Breakfast: Scrambled Tofu with Spinach and Tomatoes
- Lunch: Zucchini Noodles with Pesto and Cherry Tomatoes
- Dinner: Turkey and Vegetable Stir-Fry

Day 7:
- Breakfast: Energizing Quinoa Breakfast Bowl
- Lunch: Lemon Herb Grilled Chicken Salad
- Dinner: Baked Salmon with Dill and Lemon

Week 2:

Day 8:
- Breakfast: Blueberry Almond Smoothie
- Lunch: Quinoa and Roasted Vegetable Buddha Bowl
- Dinner: Eggplant and Chickpea Curry

Day 9:
- Breakfast: Scrambled Tofu with Spinach and Tomatoes
- Lunch: Zucchini Noodles with Pesto and Cherry Tomatoes
- Dinner: Turkey and Vegetable Stir-Fry

Day 10:
- Breakfast: Energizing Quinoa Breakfast Bowl
- Lunch: Lemon Herb Grilled Chicken Salad
- Dinner: Baked Salmon with Dill and Lemon

Day 11:
- Breakfast: Blueberry Almond Smoothie
- Lunch: Quinoa and Roasted Vegetable Buddha Bowl
- Dinner: Eggplant and Chickpea Curry

Day 12:
- Breakfast: Scrambled Tofu with Spinach and Tomatoes
- Lunch: Zucchini Noodles with Pesto and Cherry Tomatoes
- Dinner: Turkey and Vegetable Stir-Fry

Day 13:
- Breakfast: Energizing Quinoa Breakfast Bowl

- Lunch: Lemon Herb Grilled Chicken Salad
- Dinner: Baked Salmon with Dill and Lemon

Day 14:
- Breakfast: Blueberry Almond Smoothie
- Lunch: Quinoa and Roasted Vegetable Buddha Bowl
- Dinner: Eggplant and Chickpea Curry

Week 3:

Day 15:
- Breakfast: Scrambled Tofu with Spinach and Tomatoes
- Lunch: Zucchini Noodles with Pesto and Cherry Tomatoes
- Dinner: Turkey and Vegetable Stir-Fry

Day 16:
- Breakfast: Energizing Quinoa Breakfast Bowl
- Lunch: Lemon Herb Grilled Chicken Salad
- Dinner: Baked Salmon with Dill and Lemon

Day 17:
- Breakfast: Blueberry Almond Smoothie
- Lunch: Quinoa and Roasted Vegetable Buddha Bowl
- Dinner: Eggplant and Chickpea Curry

Day 18:
- Breakfast: Scrambled Tofu with Spinach and Tomatoes
- Lunch: Zucchini Noodles with Pesto and Cherry Tomatoes
- Dinner: Turkey and Vegetable Stir-Fry

Day 19:
- Breakfast: Energizing Quinoa Breakfast Bowl
- Lunch: Lemon Herb Grilled Chicken Salad
- Dinner: Baked Salmon with Dill and Lemon

Day 20:
- Breakfast: Blueberry Almond Smoothie
- Lunch: Quinoa and Roasted Vegetable Buddha Bowl
- Dinner: Eggplant and Chickpea Curry

Day 21:
- Breakfast: Scrambled Tofu with Spinach and Tomatoes
- Lunch: Zucchini Noodles with Pesto and Cherry Tomatoes
- Dinner: Turkey and Vegetable Stir-Fry

Week 4:

Day 22:
- Breakfast: Energizing Quinoa Breakfast Bowl
- Lunch: Lemon Herb Grilled Chicken Salad
- Dinner: Baked Salmon with Dill and Lemon

Day 23:
- Breakfast: Blueberry Almond Smoothie
- Lunch: Quinoa and Roasted Vegetable Buddha Bowl
- Dinner: Eggplant and Chickpea Curry

Day 24:
- Breakfast: Scrambled Tofu with Spinach and Tomatoes
- Lunch: Zucchini Noodles with Pesto and Cherry Tomatoes
- Dinner: Turkey and Vegetable Stir-Fry

Day 25:
- Breakfast: Energizing Quinoa Breakfast Bowl
- Lunch: Lemon Herb Grilled Chicken Salad
- Dinner: Baked Salmon with Dill and Lemon

Day 26:
- Breakfast: Blueberry Almond Smoothie
- Lunch: Quinoa and Roasted Vegetable Buddha Bowl
- Dinner: Eggplant and Chickpea Curry

Day 27:
- Breakfast: Scrambled Tofu with Spinach and Tomatoes
- Lunch: Zucchini Noodles with Pesto and Cherry Tomatoes
- Dinner: Turkey and Vegetable Stir-Fry

Day 28:
- Breakfast: Energizing Quinoa Breakfast Bowl
- Lunch: Lemon Herb Grilled Chicken Salad
- Dinner: Baked Salmon with Dill and Lemon

Chapter 8: Symptom Management

Tailoring Your Diet to Manage Pelvic Pain, Bloating, and Dysmenorrhea

Living with endometriosis involves navigating various symptoms that can impact daily life. This chapter focuses on tailoring your diet to alleviate specific symptoms such as pelvic pain, bloating, and dysmenorrhea. The Low FODMAP approach plays a crucial role in managing these symptoms, as certain foods can either trigger or alleviate discomfort. Here's how you can adapt your diet for symptom relief:

Managing Pelvic Pain:

1. Incorporate Anti-Inflammatory Foods: Include foods rich in omega-3 fatty acids, such as fatty fish (salmon, mackerel), flaxseeds, and walnuts, to help reduce inflammation associated with pelvic pain.

2. Turmeric and Ginger: Add these anti-inflammatory spices to your meals. Consider turmeric tea or incorporating ginger into stir-fries for their potential pain-relieving properties.

3. Hydration: Ensure adequate hydration to maintain overall health and support the body's natural processes. Herbal teas and water can be soothing.

Alleviating Bloating:

1. Low FODMAP Choices: Stick to low FODMAP foods to minimize gas production and bloating. The cookbook's recipes are crafted with this in mind, offering flavorful meals without triggering discomfort.

2. Digestive Enzymes: Consider incorporating digestive enzymes before meals to aid in the breakdown of certain foods, potentially reducing bloating.

3. Probiotics: Include low FODMAP probiotic-rich foods like lactose-free yogurt to support a healthy gut microbiome, which can contribute to improved digestion.

Managing Dysmenorrhea:

1. Omega-3 Fatty Acids: Continue to emphasize foods rich in omega-3 fatty acids, which may help reduce inflammation and alleviate menstrual pain.

2. Magnesium-Rich Foods: Magnesium can contribute to muscle relaxation. Include magnesium-rich foods such as leafy greens, nuts, and seeds.

3. Gentle Exercise: Incorporate gentle exercises like yoga or walking into your routine, which may help manage pain associated with dysmenorrhea.

Personalized Approach:

1. Keep a Food Diary: Track your diet alongside symptom flare-ups to identify potential trigger foods. This personalized approach can help you understand your body's unique responses.

2. Consult with a Dietitian: Consider consulting with a registered dietitian specializing in endometriosis to create a personalized nutrition plan tailored to your specific needs and preferences.

3. Mindful Eating: Practice mindful eating to foster a positive relationship with food. Pay attention to how your body responds to different meals and adjust accordingly.

Empower Yourself Through Nutrition

By understanding how certain foods impact your symptoms and incorporating the principles outlined in this chapter, you can empower yourself to take an active role in managing pelvic pain, bloating, and dysmenorrhea. The recipes in this cookbook are designed to support your journey toward digestive wellness and overall well-being.

Addressing Infertility Concerns through Nutrition

For individuals facing endometriosis-related fertility challenges, nutrition plays a crucial role in supporting reproductive health and overall well-being. This chapter focuses on how specific dietary choices can contribute to managing infertility concerns associated with endometriosis.

Nutrient-Rich Foods for Reproductive Health:

1. Folate-Rich Foods: Incorporate foods rich in folate, such as leafy greens, citrus fruits, and legumes, which are essential for preconception and early pregnancy.

2. Omega-3 Fatty Acids: Emphasize foods high in omega-3 fatty acids, like fatty fish, flaxseeds, and walnuts, which may support reproductive function and improve fertility.

3. Antioxidant-Rich Choices: Opt for a variety of colorful fruits and vegetables to ensure a broad spectrum of antioxidants. Berries, tomatoes, and bell peppers are excellent choices.

Balancing Hormones through Diet:

1. Healthy Fats: Include sources of healthy fats like avocados, olive oil, and nuts to support hormone production and balance.

2. Lean Proteins: Choose lean protein sources, such as poultry, fish, and tofu, to provide essential amino acids crucial for hormone synthesis.

3. Whole Grains: Opt for whole grains like quinoa and brown rice, which offer complex carbohydrates and fiber that may help stabilize blood sugar levels and hormonal balance.

Supporting Gut Health:

1. Probiotics: Incorporate low FODMAP probiotic-rich foods to promote a healthy gut microbiome, which is linked to improved fertility.

2. Fiber-Rich Foods: Include fiber from fruits, vegetables, and whole grains to support digestive health, which plays a role in overall well-being and fertility.

Lifestyle Factors:

1. Maintain a Healthy Weight: Achieving and maintaining a healthy weight is essential for reproductive health. A balanced diet and regular exercise contribute to overall well-being.

2. Stay Hydrated: Proper hydration supports overall health and can positively influence reproductive functions.

Personalized Approach:

1. Consultation with a Specialist: If fertility concerns persist, consider consulting with a reproductive specialist or fertility nutritionist to create a personalized plan tailored to your unique needs.

2. Mind-Body Practices: Incorporate stress-reducing practices such as yoga, meditation, or deep-breathing exercises, as stress management is integral to reproductive health.

Fertility-Focused Nutrition

While no diet can guarantee fertility success, adopting a nutrient-rich, balanced diet tailored to your individual needs can contribute to overall reproductive health. The recipes in this cookbook are crafted with these principles in mind, supporting your journey toward improved well-being and fertility.

Chapter 9: Tips for Success

Incorporating Low FODMAP Principles into Your Lifestyle

Adopting a Low FODMAP lifestyle is not just about following a temporary diet but embracing a long-term approach to support digestive wellness and manage endometriosis symptoms. This chapter provides practical tips for seamlessly incorporating Low FODMAP principles into your daily life.

1. Educate Yourself:
   - Take the time to understand the basics of the Low FODMAP approach. Familiarize yourself with high and low FODMAP foods to make informed choices.

2. Gradual Implementation:
   - Introduce Low FODMAP principles gradually into your diet. This allows you to assess your body's response and identify trigger foods.

3. Variety is Key:
   - Explore a variety of Low FODMAP recipes from this cookbook. A diverse and balanced diet ensures you receive a spectrum of nutrients.

4. Meal Prep and Planning:
   - Plan your meals in advance and incorporate meal-prep strategies. This minimizes stress and makes it easier to stick to your dietary goals.

5. Label Reading:
   - Develop the habit of reading food labels to identify potential FODMAPs. Many packaged foods may contain hidden ingredients that could trigger symptoms.

6. Communication:
   - Communicate your dietary needs with friends, family, and colleagues. This ensures a supportive environment, especially during social gatherings.

7. Stay Hydrated:
   - Hydration is essential for overall health and digestion. Drink plenty of water throughout the day to support your body's natural processes.

8. Mindful Eating:
   - Practice mindful eating by paying attention to hunger and fullness cues. This can help prevent overeating and enhance your connection with food.

9. Recipe Adaptations:
   - Feel free to adapt recipes to suit your preferences and dietary needs. Substitute ingredients as necessary, keeping in mind the principles of the Low FODMAP approach.

10. Seek Professional Guidance:
   - If needed, consult with a registered dietitian specializing in the Low FODMAP diet. A professional can provide personalized guidance and support.

11. Explore Low FODMAP Brands:
   - Discover Low FODMAP-friendly brands for convenience. Many specialty products are available, making it easier to maintain your dietary choices.

12. Mind-Body Connection:
   - Recognize the connection between stress and digestive symptoms. Incorporate stress-management techniques such as yoga, meditation, or deep-breathing exercises.

13. Celebrate Progress:
   - Celebrate small victories along your journey. Recognize the positive changes and improvements in your digestive wellness.

Staying Motivated and Enjoying the Journey

Embarking on a journey to adopt a Low FODMAP lifestyle can be transformative, but like any change, it requires motivation and a positive mindset. This chapter provides insights and strategies to help you stay motivated and savor the experience of embracing a Low FODMAP way of life.

1. Set Realistic Goals:
   - Establish achievable and realistic goals for your Low FODMAP journey. Break down larger goals into smaller, manageable steps.

2. Celebrate Small Wins:
   - Acknowledge and celebrate every achievement, no matter how small. Whether it's trying a new recipe or successfully navigating a social event, these victories matter.

3. Create a Support System:
   - Surround yourself with a supportive network of friends, family, or fellow individuals on a Low FODMAP journey. Share experiences, challenges, and triumphs.

4. Variety is Exciting:
   - Embrace the excitement of trying new Low FODMAP recipes. The cookbook offers a diverse range of dishes to keep your meals interesting and satisfying.

5. Document Your Progress:
   - Keep a journal to document your experiences, including how your body responds to different foods. Reflecting on progress can be a powerful motivator.

6. Mindful Eating Practices:
   - Engage in mindful eating. Savor each bite, appreciate the flavors, and be present during meals. This fosters a positive relationship with food.

7. Reward Yourself:

- Incorporate rewards for achieving milestones. Treat yourself to something enjoyable, whether it's a relaxing activity, a favorite hobby, or a special treat within your dietary restrictions.

8. Stay Informed:

- Stay updated on new Low FODMAP research, recipes, and resources. Knowledge empowers you to make informed choices and stay engaged in your journey.

9. Find Joy in Cooking:

- Rediscover the joy of cooking. Experiment with herbs, spices, and Low FODMAP ingredients to create delicious and satisfying meals.

10. Mind-Body Connection:

- Cultivate a positive mind-body connection. Engage in activities that bring you joy, reduce stress, and contribute to your overall well-being.

11. Adapt and Learn:

- Embrace a mindset of continuous learning and adaptation. As you discover what works best for your body, remain flexible and open to adjustments.

12. Share Your Journey:

- Share your Low FODMAP journey with others. Your experiences may inspire and motivate those facing similar challenges.

13. Enjoy the Process:

- Remember that the journey itself is valuable. Enjoy the process of discovering new flavors, understanding your body, and taking steps toward improved well-being.

Conclusion

Your Path to Wellness

Congratulations on embarking on this journey toward improved well-being through the Low FODMAP Endometriosis Cookbook. As you conclude this exploration of nutritious recipes, practical tips, and holistic guidance, it's essential to reflect on your unique path to wellness.

Celebrating Achievements:
Take a moment to acknowledge the progress you've made. Whether you've discovered new favorite recipes, successfully navigated social events, or found relief from specific symptoms, each achievement is a step toward your overall wellness.

Mind-Body Connection:
Recognize the interconnectedness of your mind and body. The choices you make in the kitchen, your approach to mindful eating, and your engagement in stress-reducing practices contribute to a harmonious mind-body connection.

Empowering Choices:
You've gained the knowledge to make empowered choices about your diet. By understanding the principles of the Low FODMAP approach, you've equipped yourself with the tools to manage symptoms and support your digestive wellness.

A Sustainable Lifestyle:
Consider the sustainability of the changes you've implemented. The recipes provided in this cookbook are not just a temporary fix but a foundation for a sustainable, long-term approach to nutrition and well-being.

Continuous Learning:
Wellness is a dynamic journey that involves continuous learning. Stay curious, explore new recipes, and remain open to adapting your approach based on your evolving understanding of your body and its needs.

Building Resilience:
Endometriosis may present unique challenges, but your journey is a testament to your resilience. Continue to navigate this path with courage, adaptability, and the confidence that comes from understanding and honoring your body.

Supporting Others:
Your experiences can be a source of inspiration and support for others facing similar challenges. Share your journey, insights, and the positive impact of the Low FODMAP lifestyle with your community.